MommyHooray Presents:

# Default Parent

*When Responsibility Quietly Finds One Person*

by MommyHooray

MommyHooray Presents: Default Parent
by MommyHooray



Written and published under the pen name MommyHooray.
Illustrations created using digital illustration tools.

Printed in the United States of America.

ISBN: 978-1-972071-41-0



For more stories and updates, visit:
https://sites.google.com/view/mommyhooray

*For the ones who became the default—*

*The ones who notice, remember, and hold it all together.*
*The ones who step in, again and again, without being asked.*

*May you feel seen in all that you carry.*
*May you feel supported in ways that truly reach you.*
*May you find moments to set things down.*

*May you remember—*
*you are more than what you carry.*

With Googolplex Love,

MommyHooray ♡

You didn't decide to carry so much.
It grew slowly, quietly, over time.

You noticed what needed to be done.
You filled the gaps.
You held things together because someone had to.

The small things stacked.
They stayed.

It became familiar.
It became expected.
It became heavy.

And still, you kept going.

Because your love kept showing up.

And you're allowed to set some of it down
and still be enough.

It didn’t start as a role.

It started with remembering
one small thing that needed to be done.

Then another.

Over time, remembering became expected.
And eventually, it became yours.

What began as noticing
became the quiet way you hold things together.

One thing
became everything.

You remember what time to leave,
what can't be forgotten,
what happens if something is missed.

It runs quietly in your mind,
even when you're not thinking about it.

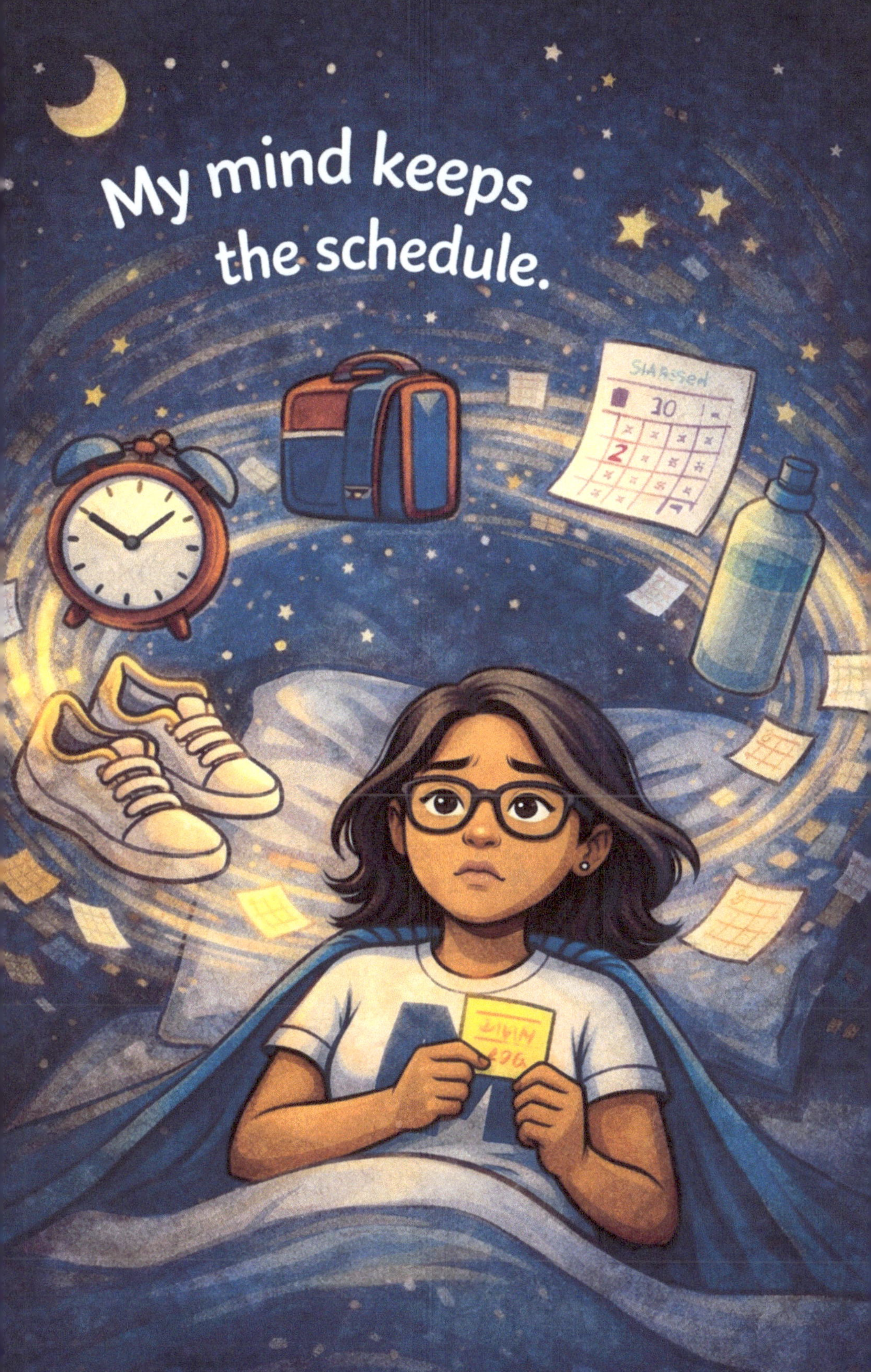
My mind keeps
the schedule.

You stepped in because it needed doing.
Because you could.
Because it felt easier than explaining.

No one handed it to you.
It simply stayed.

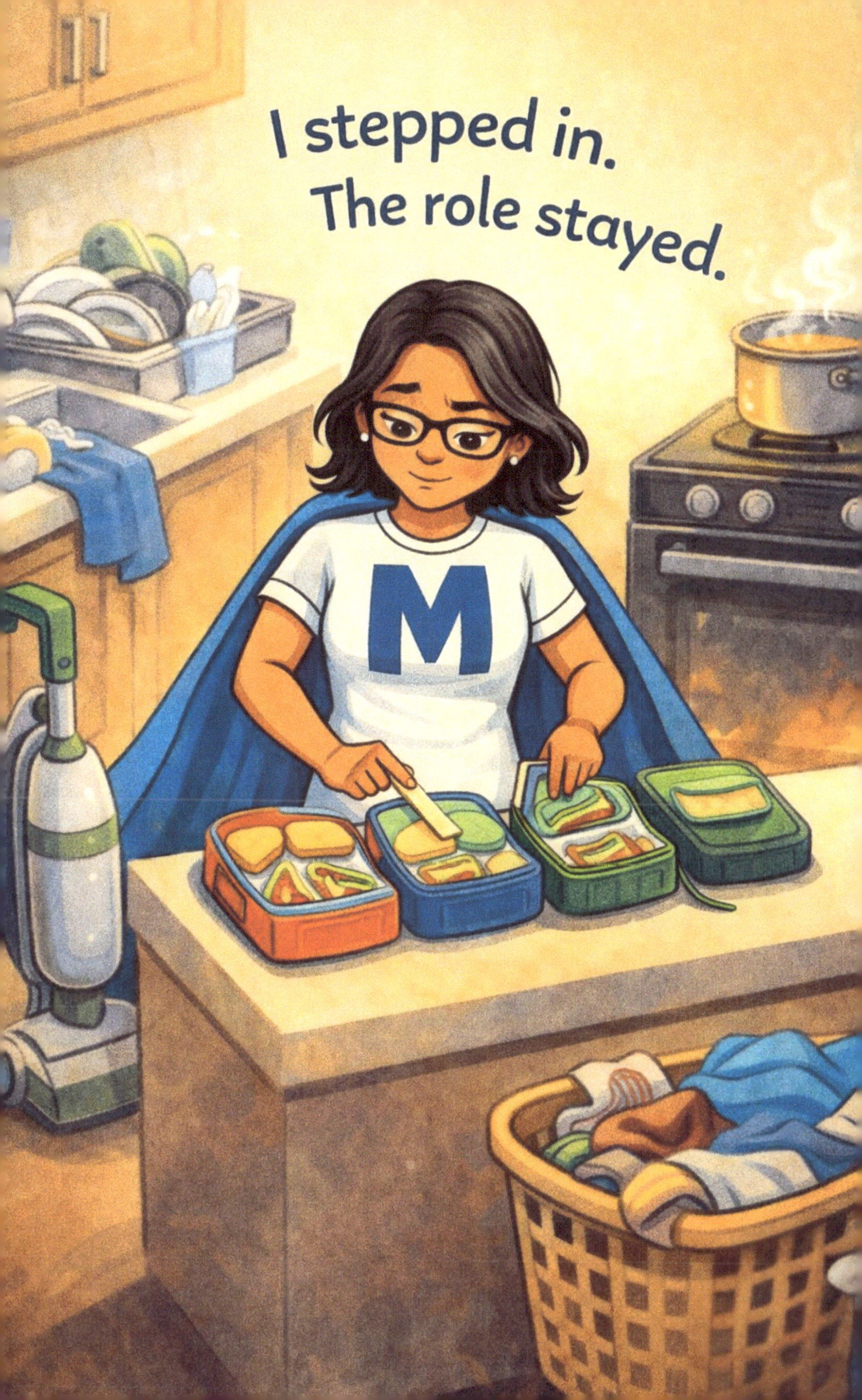
I stepped in.
The role stayed.
M

The tiredness wasn't loud.

It was constant.

The kind that lingers even after rest.

The kind that quietly follows you through the day.

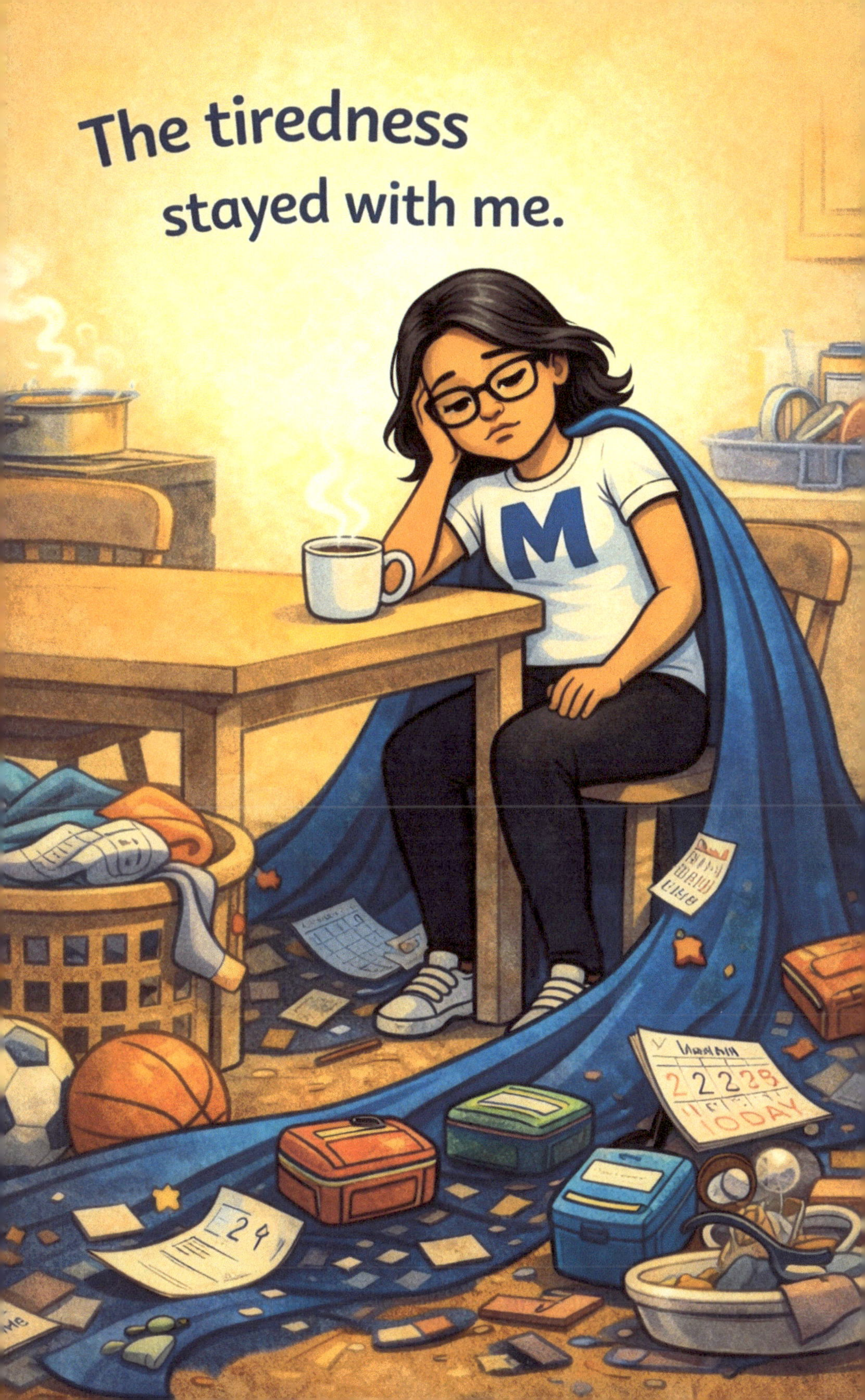

The tiredness stayed with me.

They show up and they care
about the life you're building together.

This isn't about blame.

It's about weight,
and how some of it
quietly becomes yours to hold.

Care and weight
don't always feel equal.

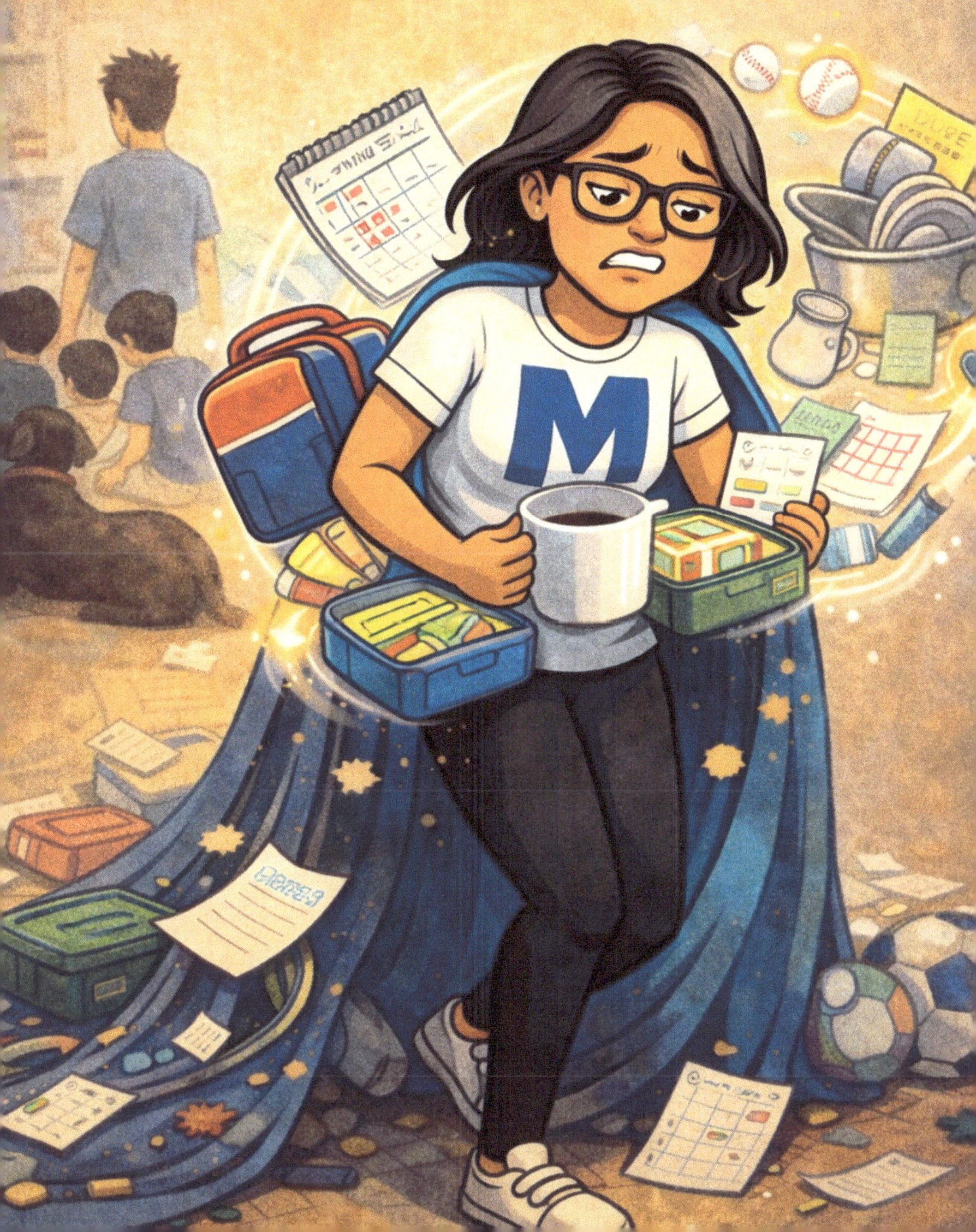

Care doesn't always mean responsibility
is shared.

Sometimes, it simply means
you're the one trusted to hold it.

And that trust...
when it rests on you for too long,
can begin to feel heavy.

Trust can become weight.

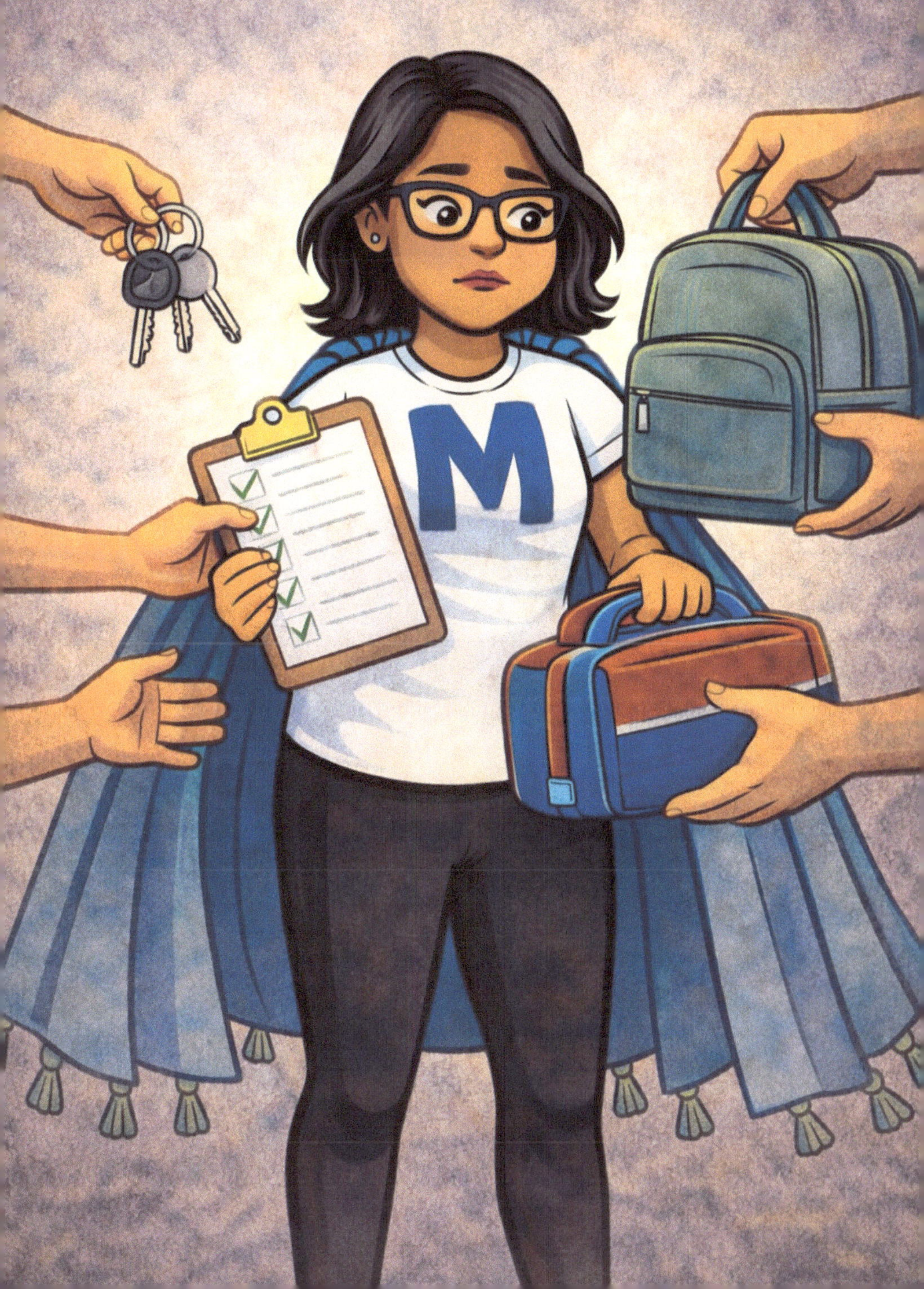

Most of the time, no one notices it happening.

Expectations settle in quietly.

Assumptions grow roots.

Nothing intentional.

Still real.

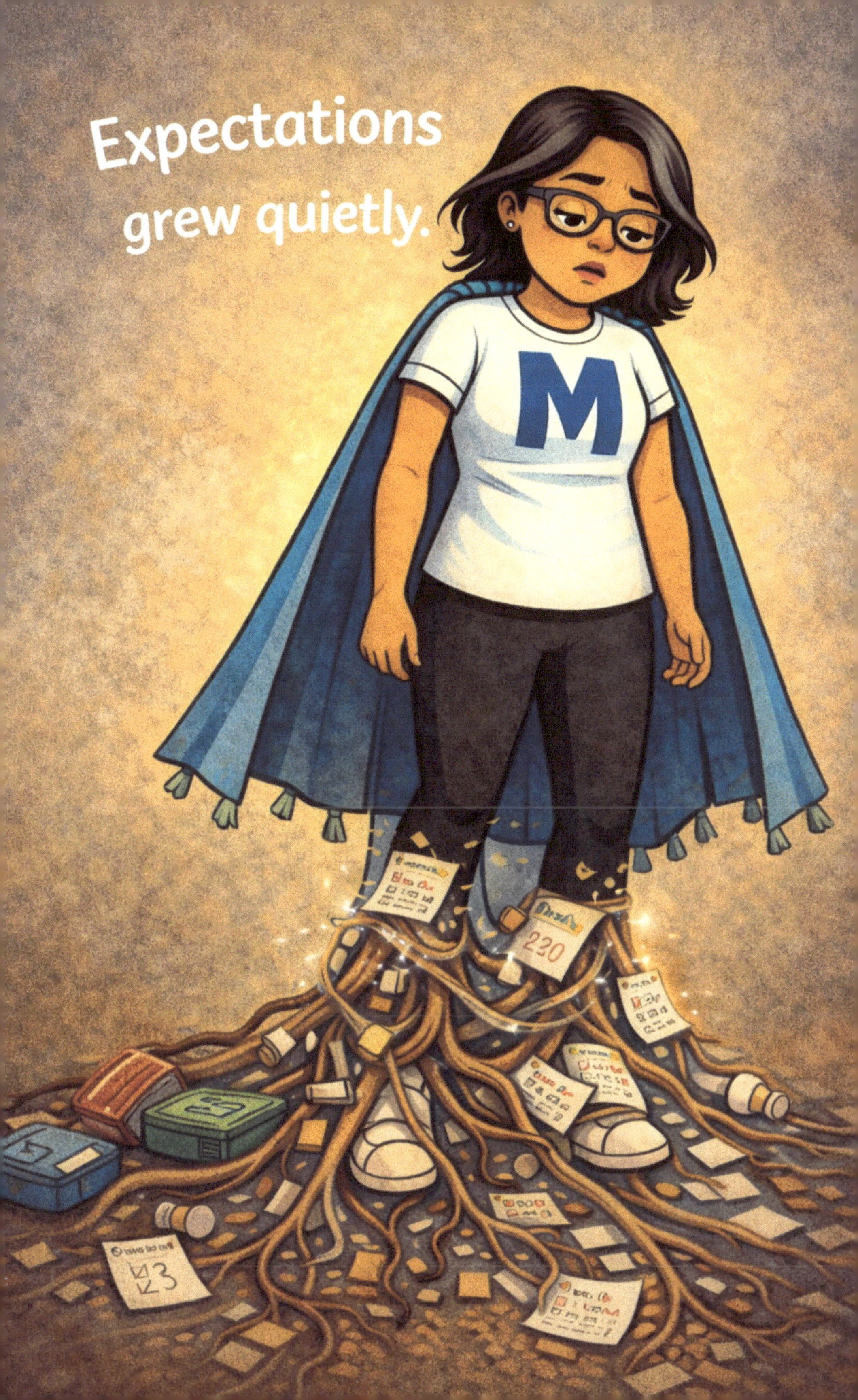
Expectations
grew quietly.

Even when love is present
and no harm was meant,
you're allowed to name
the weight you've been carrying.

That isn't blame.
It's clarity.

And sometimes,
that's the first step toward something lighter.

Naming the weight matters.

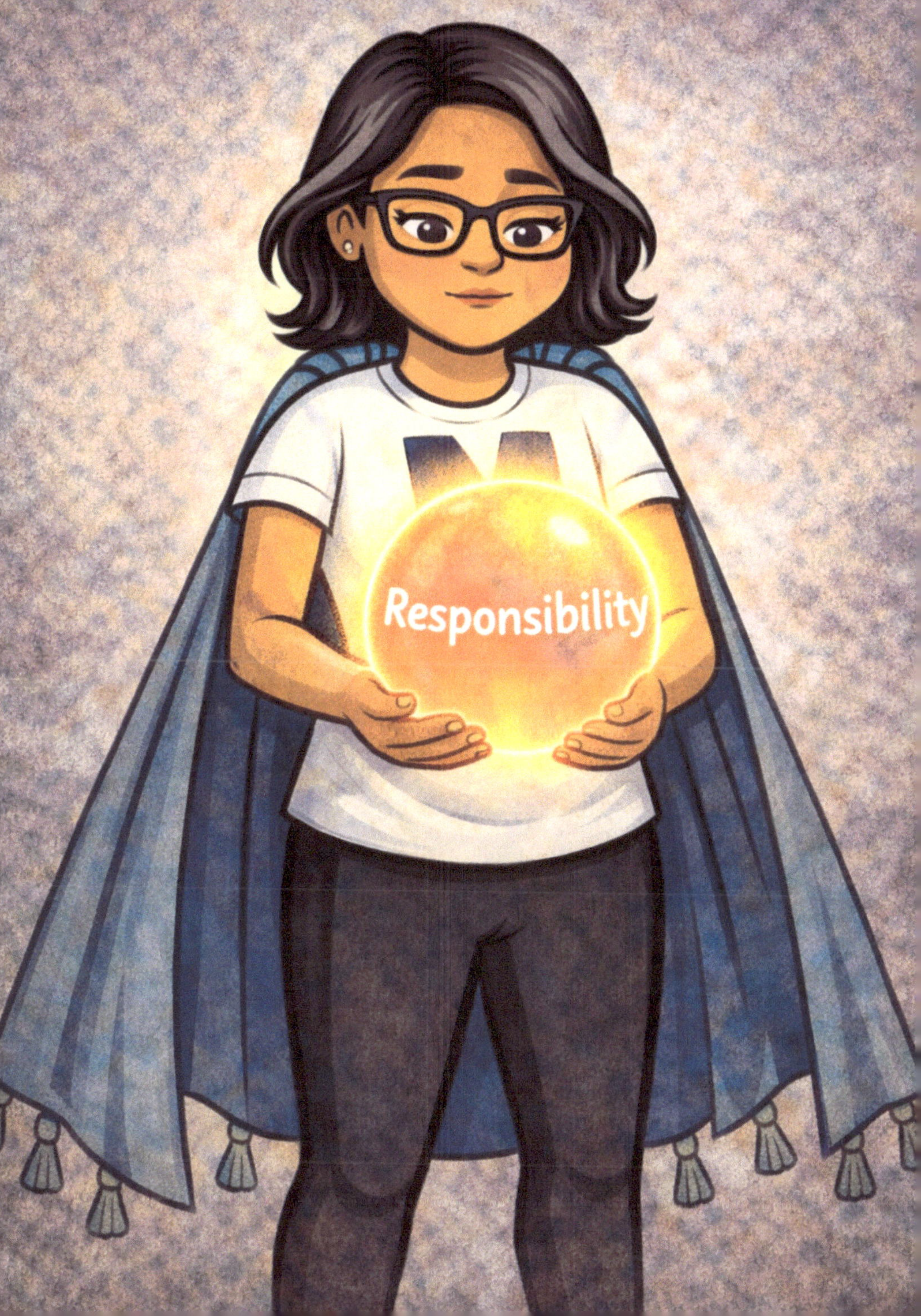

Some responsibilities don't have an end point.

They stay with you long after the moment passes.

They live in your body.

In your thoughts.

Quietly waiting in the background.

Some roles never clock out.

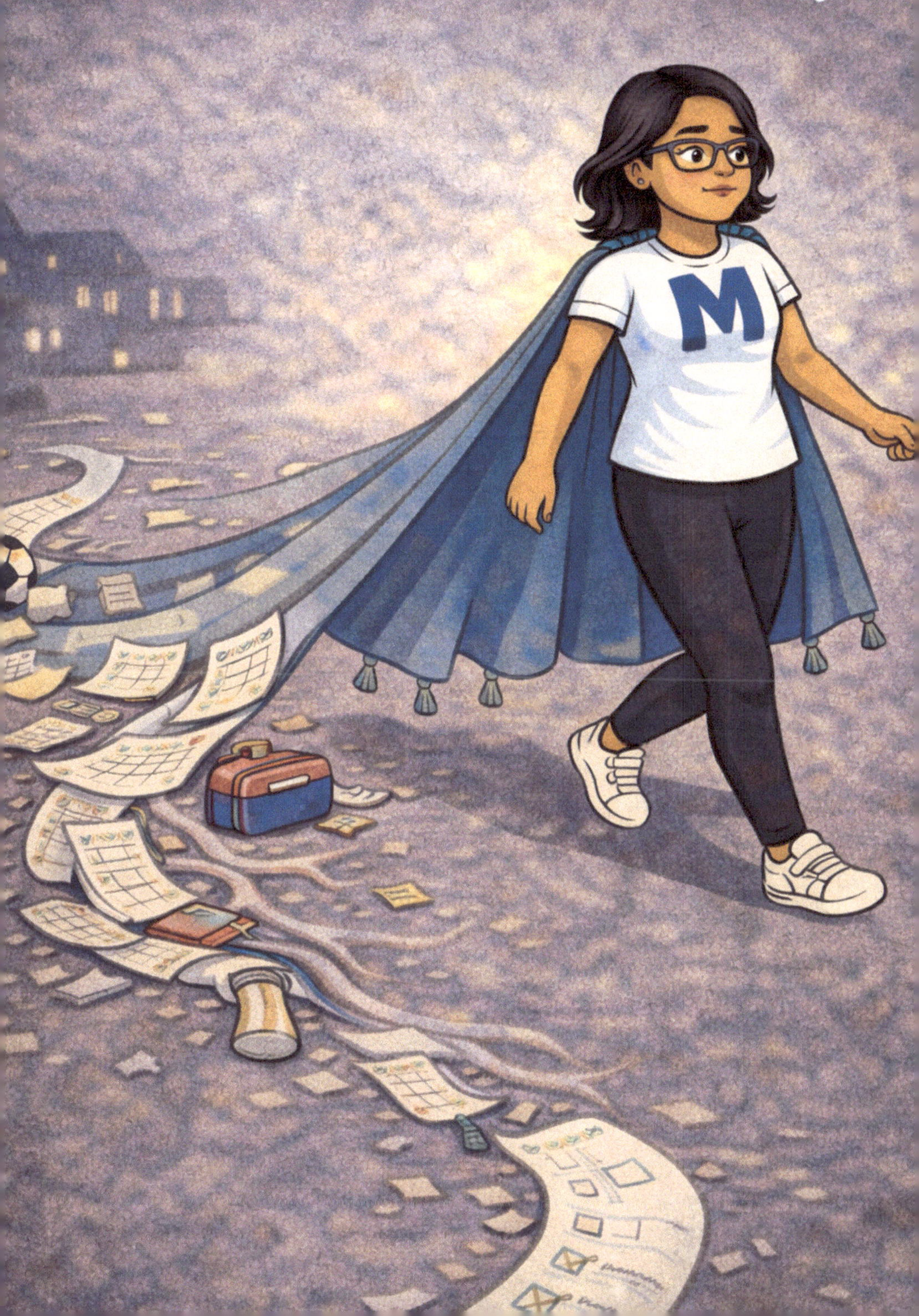

You sense what's coming before it arrives.

You prepare for what others haven't noticed yet.

You think a few steps ahead.

You consider what might be needed next.

You hold space.

You steady the moment.

You keep the day from unraveling.

I'm already reaching.

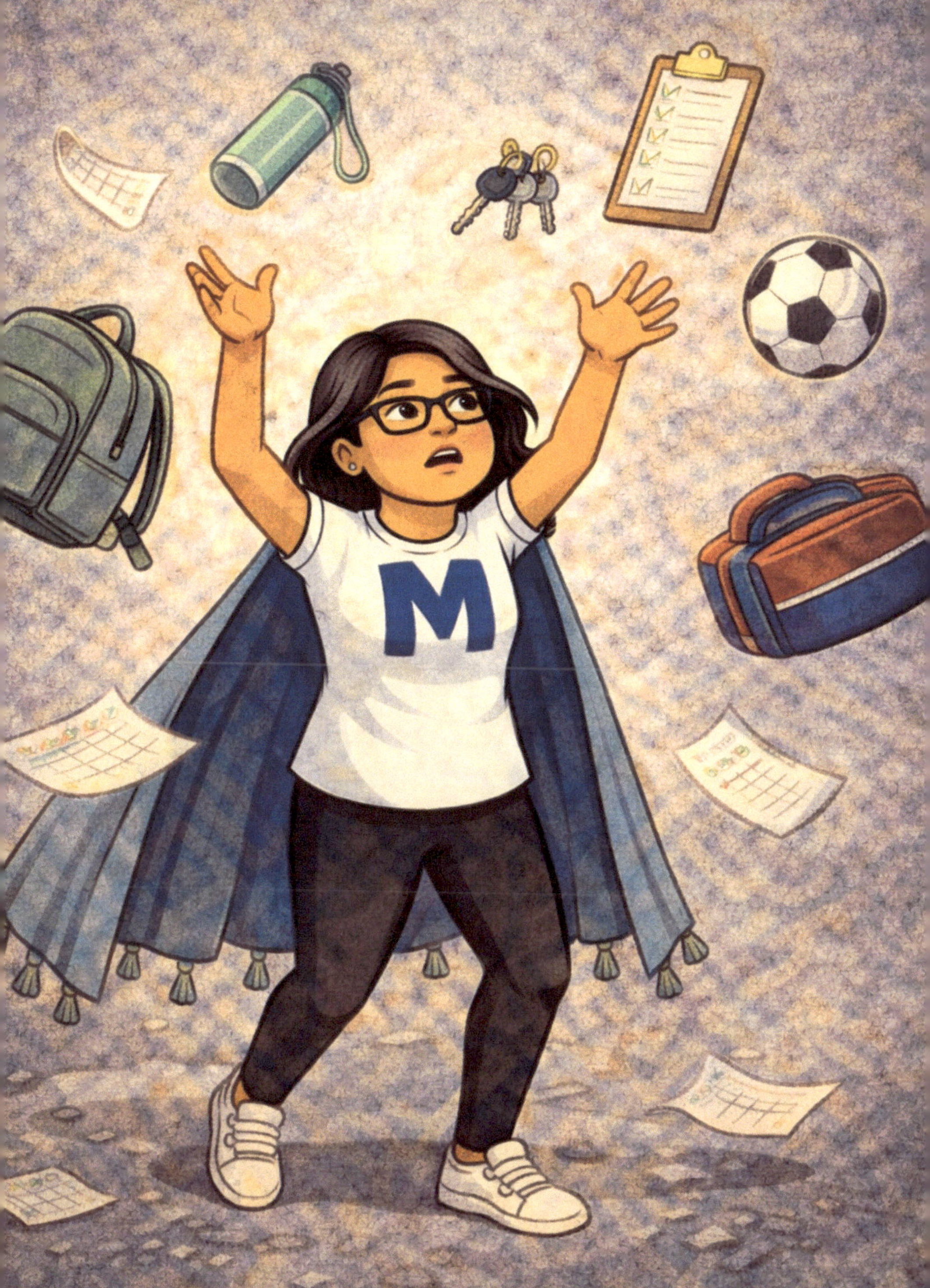

You soften the edges of conversations

before they cut too deeply.

You lower the volume when emotions begin to rise.

You keep the peace in ways that often go unseen.

You become the place

where tension has somewhere to go.

I hold the calm.

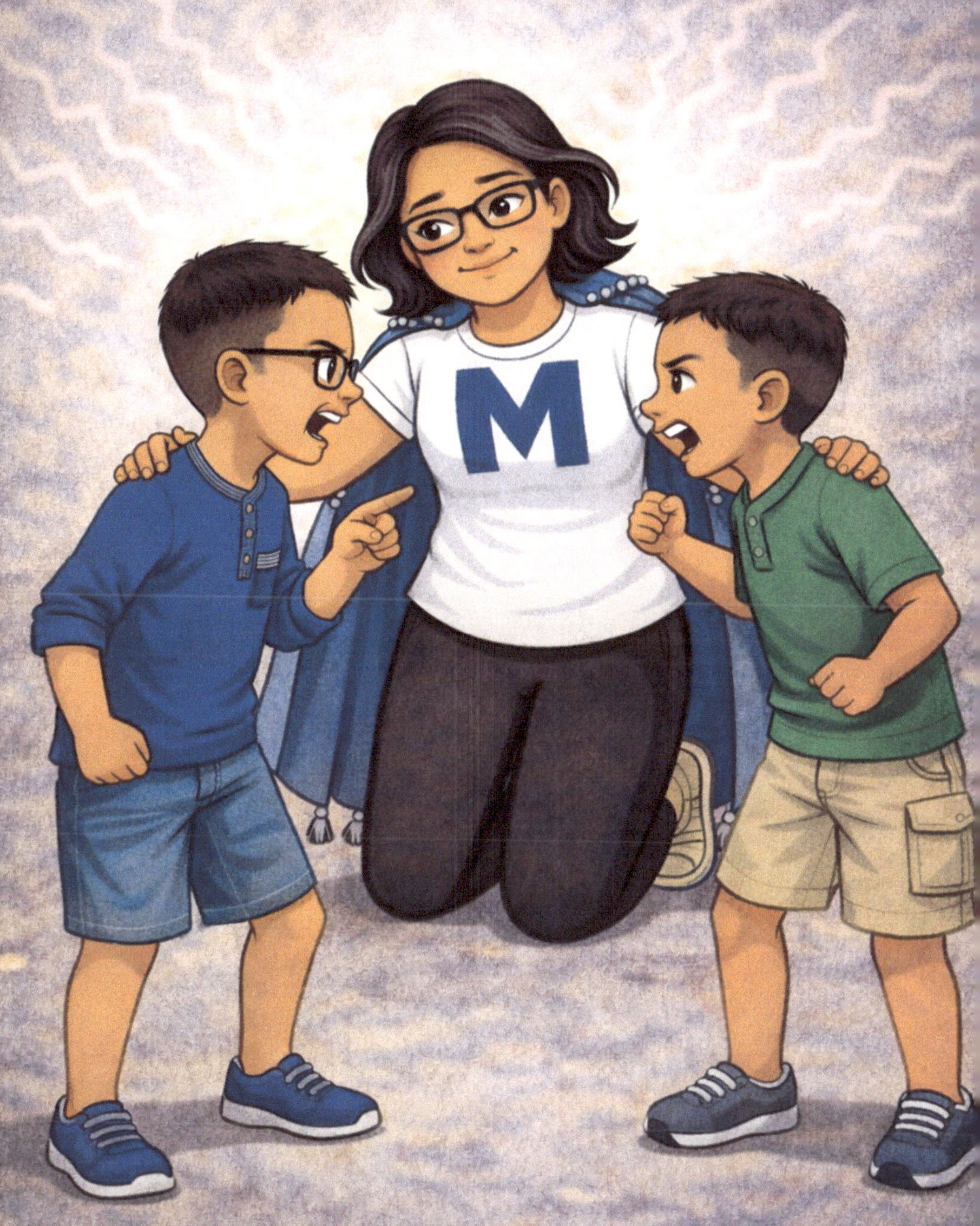

Everything passes through you.

Plans.

Emotions.

Needs.

You notice what's needed.

You remember what's coming.

You steady the moment when things feel uncertain.

You are the constant—

even when no one names it.

Everything passes through me.

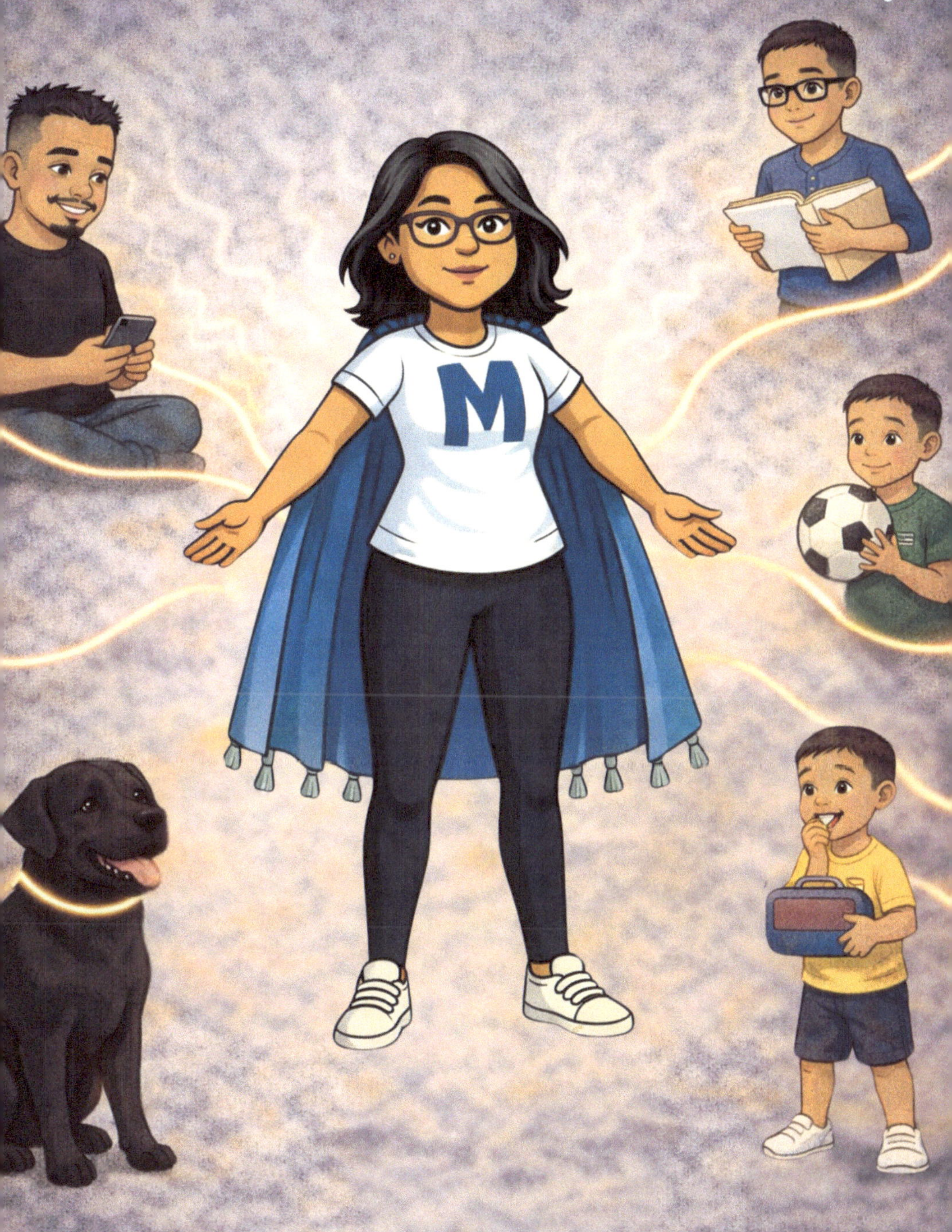

Not completely, and not all at once.

Just quietly, in small ways that add up over time.

A little less space for you.

A little more space for everyone else.

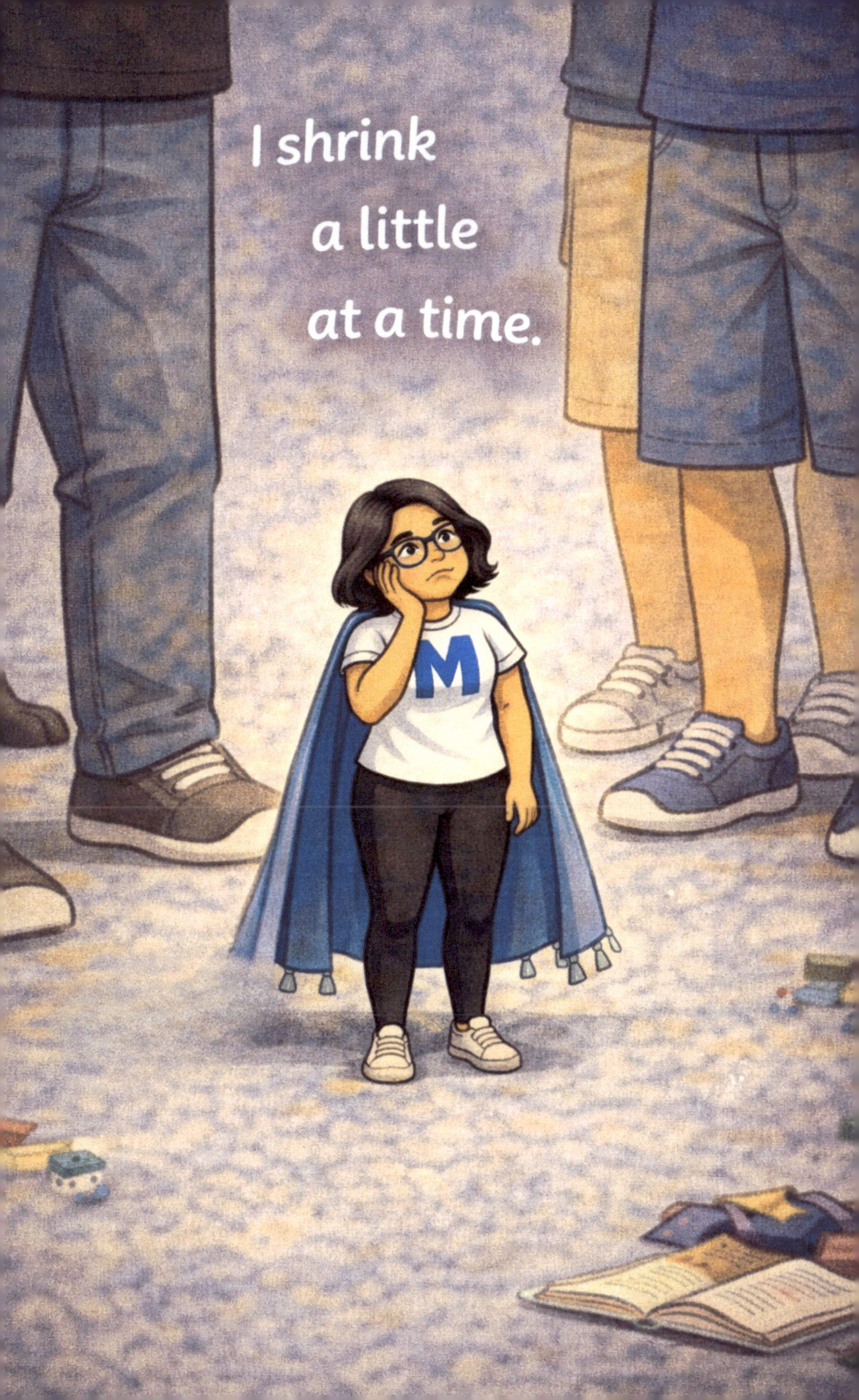
I shrink
a little
at a time.

You rest only after everything is handled,
after everyone else is okay.

And somehow, rest keeps getting postponed.

There is always something left to do,
something else that needs you first.

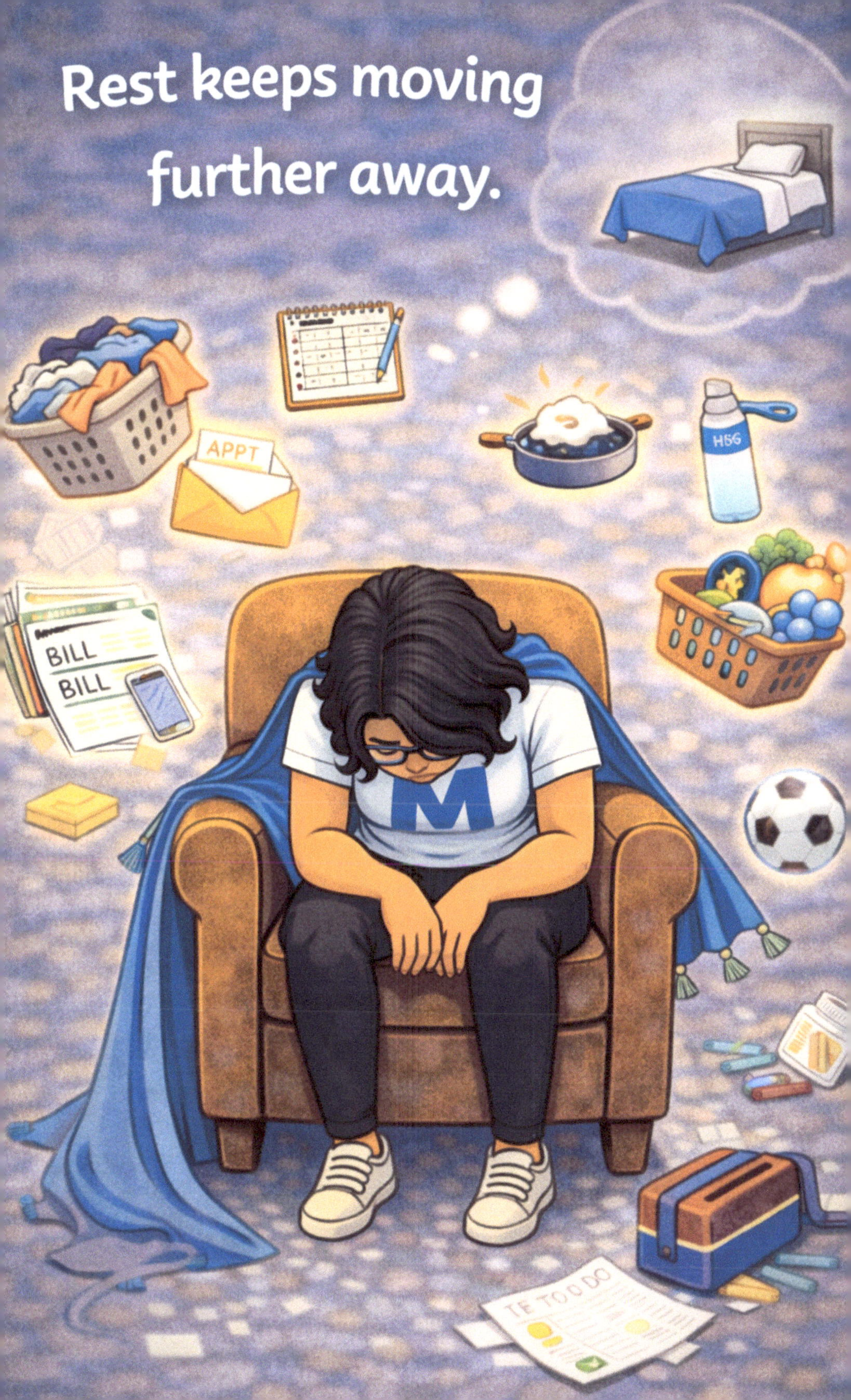
Rest keeps moving
further away.
APPT
BILL
BILL

Love does involve care, effort, and responsibility.

It asks for presence, for patience,
and for the quiet work of showing up every day.

But love was never meant
to require you to slowly disappear in the process.

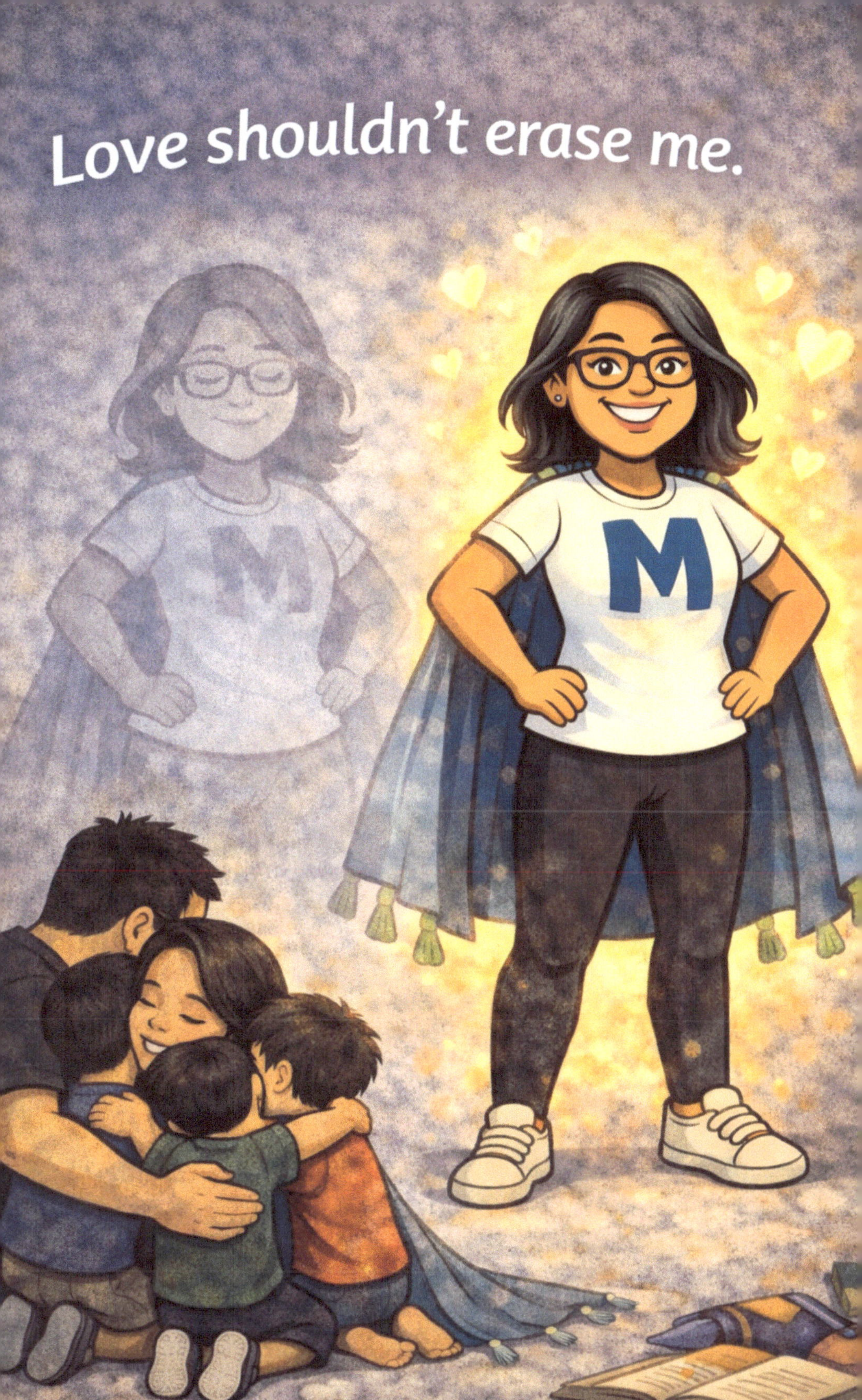
Love shouldn't erase me.
M
M

You don't need to give everything to be enough.
You were always enough already.

The love you give is meaningful.
But you were never meant to lose yourself
while giving it.

You are allowed to live,
not just hold everything together.

I was always enough.

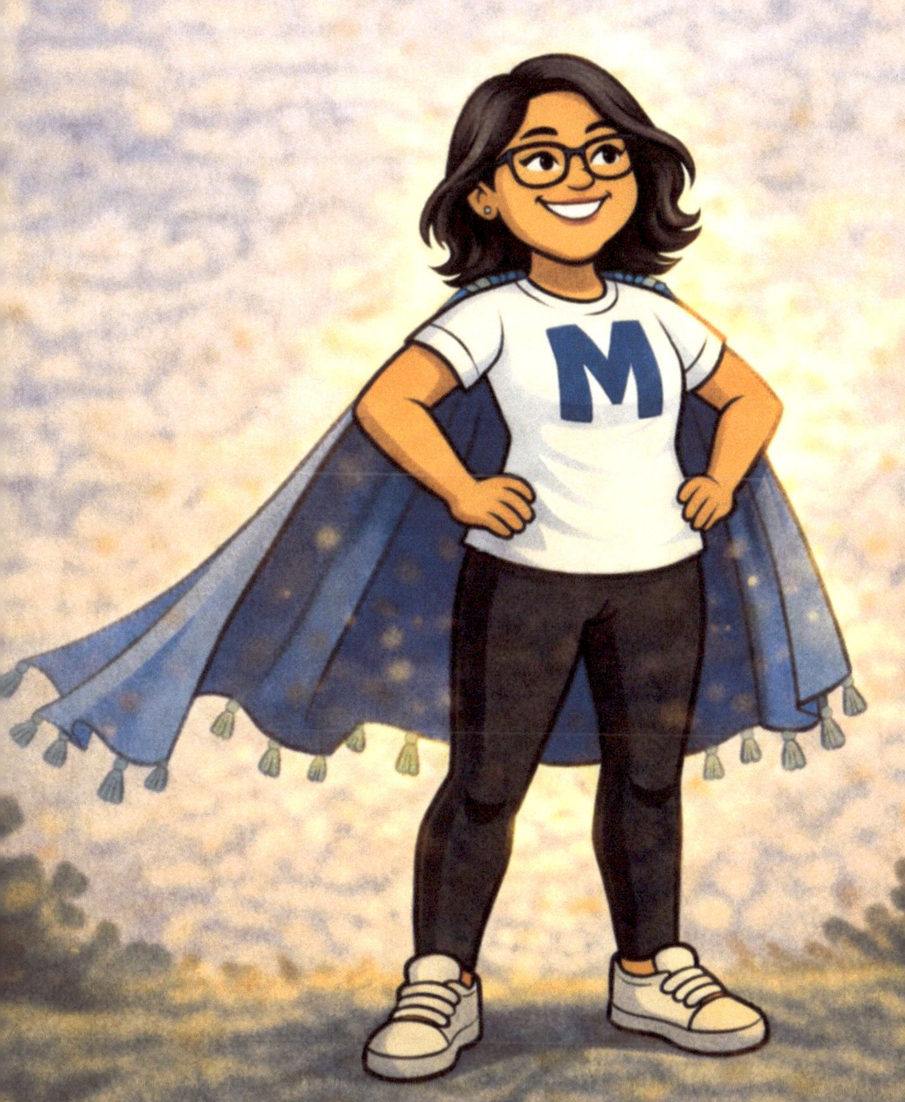

Rest doesn't require escape
from the life you've built.

It doesn't require silence
or distance from everything you love.

Rest can exist quietly right where you are.

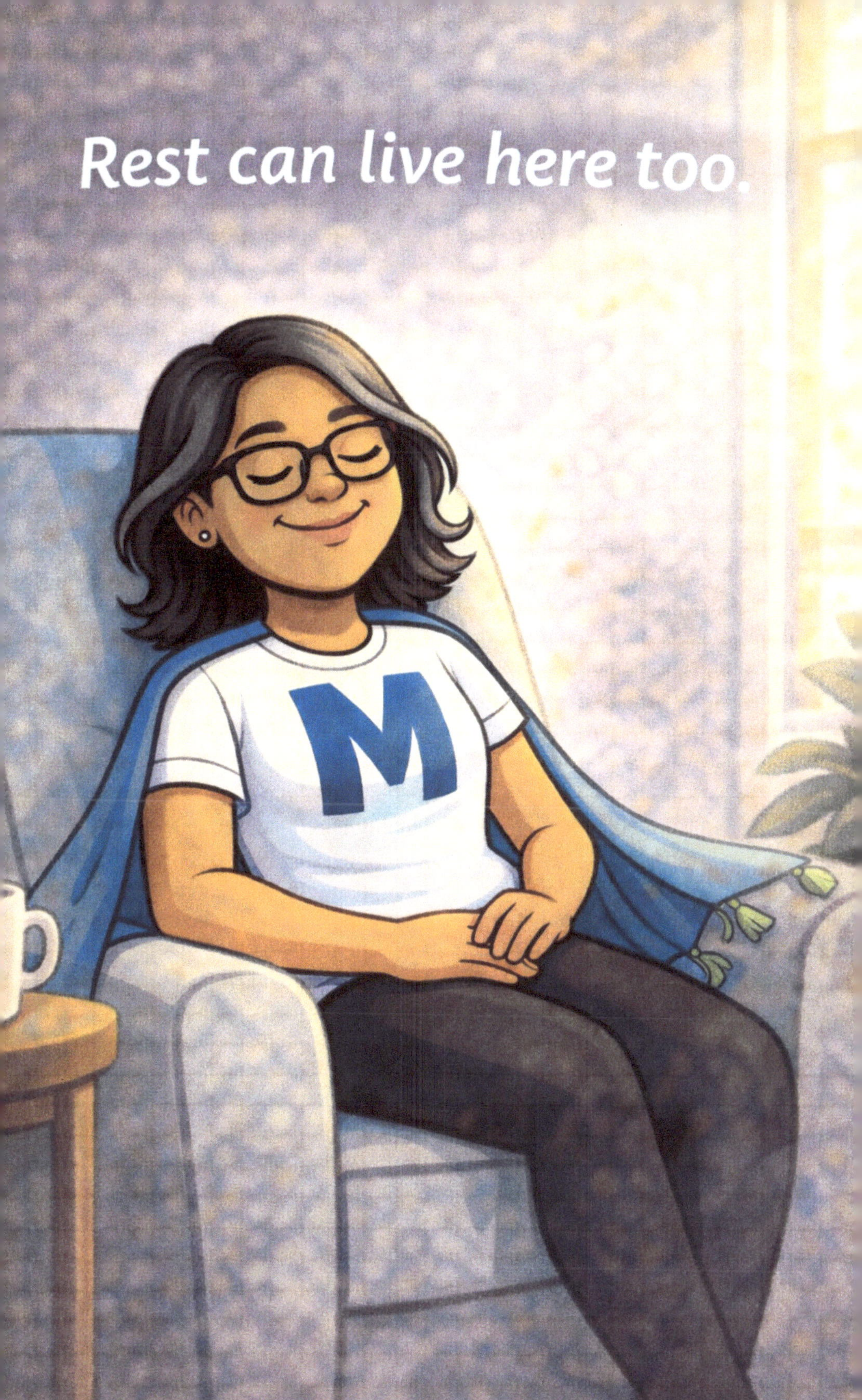
Rest can live here too.
M

You don't have to wait
until everything feels overwhelming.

Support was never meant to arrive
only when things fall apart.

You're allowed to ask sooner.
You're allowed to be supported along the way.

I'm allowed to ask.

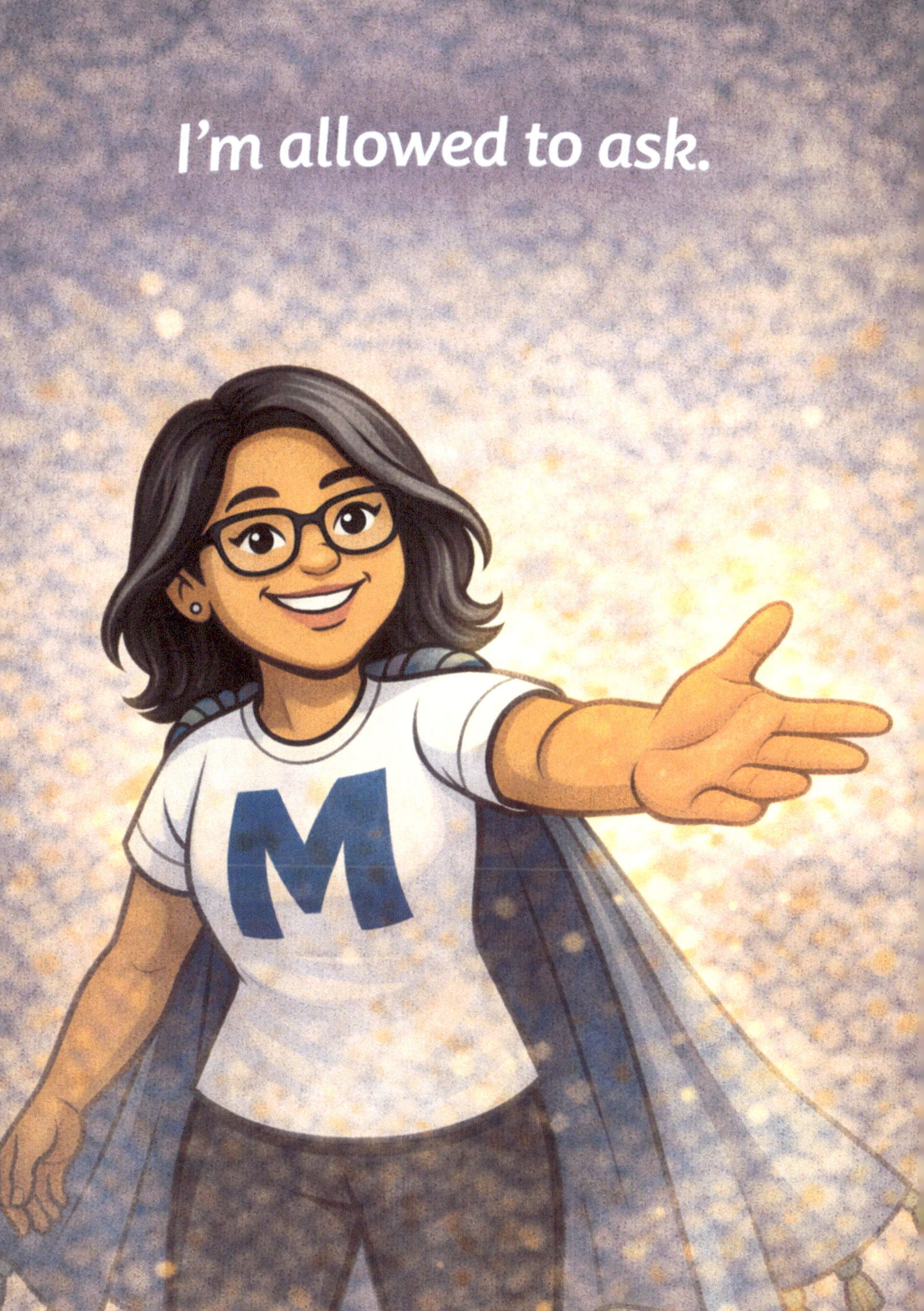

The weight you've been carrying
can be shared with others.

It can be learned and understood with time.
And little by little, it can be rebalanced.

Not perfectly,
but more gently.

The weight can be shared.

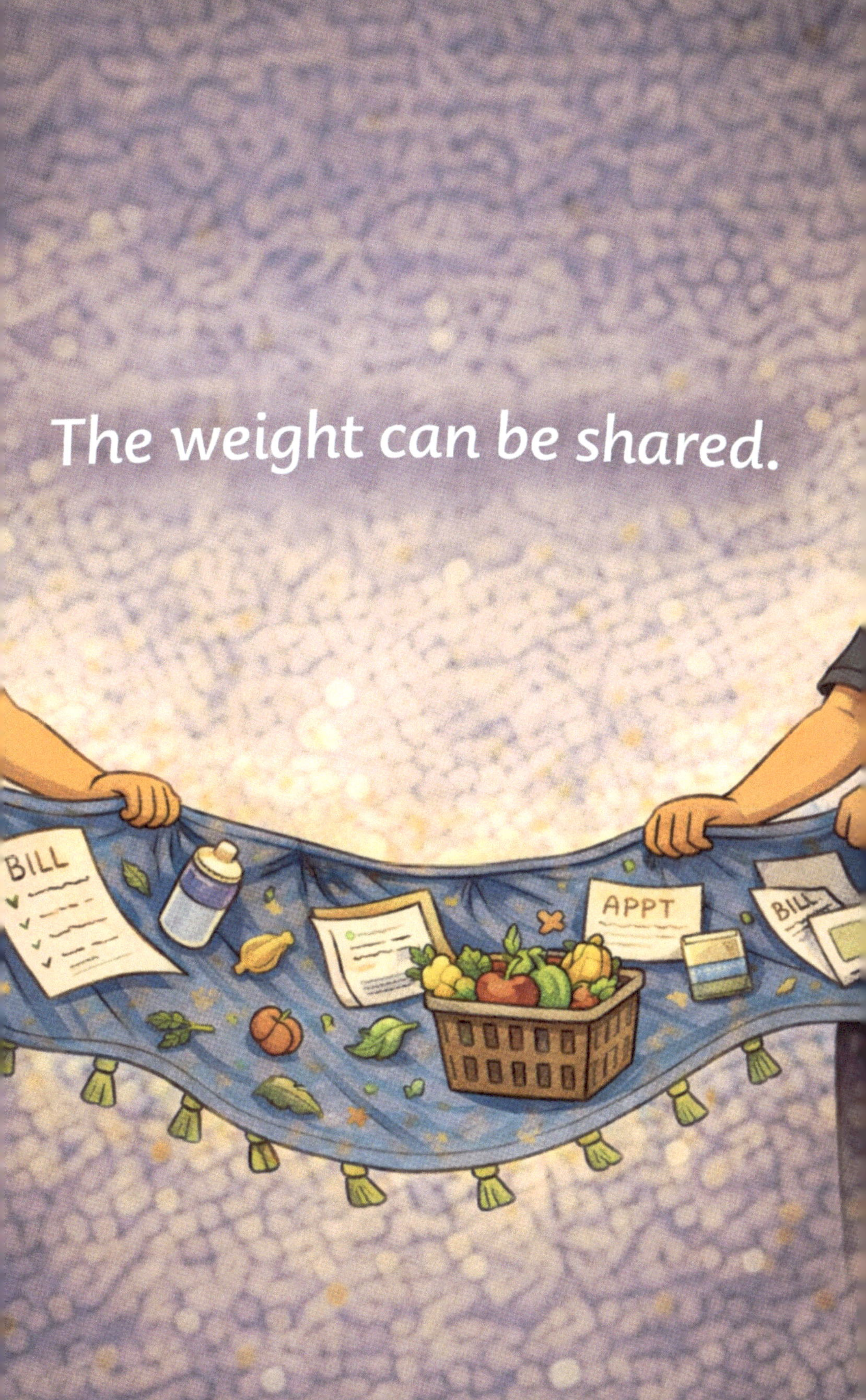

You are not just the one who carries what everyone else depends on.

You are someone who deserves care, attention, and space to rest.

You don't have to earn that.
You already deserve it.

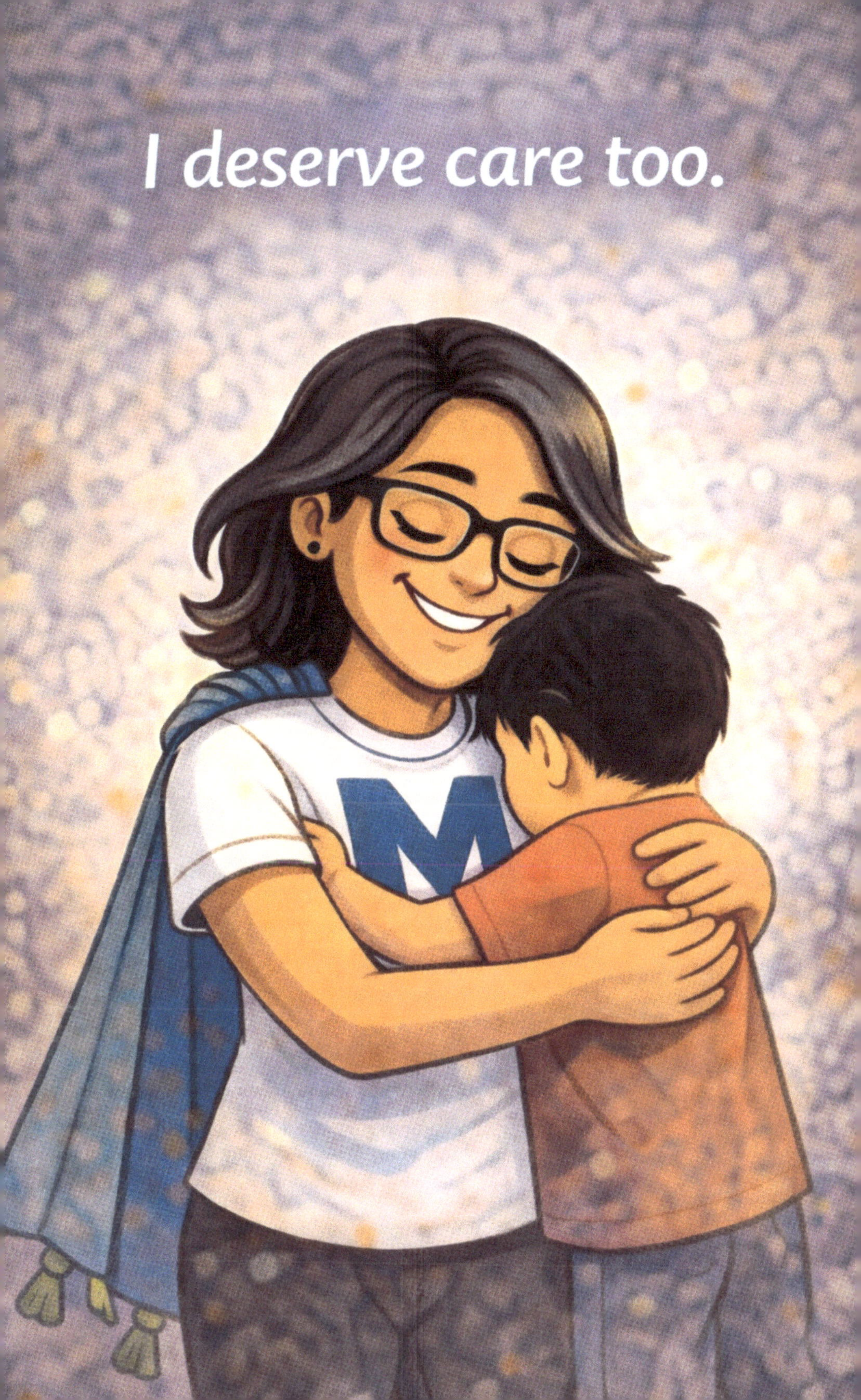
I deserve care too.
M

You don't have to hold everything to be worthy.
You don't have to stay strong all the time.

It's okay to set things down.
It's okay to let others carry some of the weight.

You are allowed to rest.
You are allowed to be supported.
You are allowed to take up space,
even without a reason.

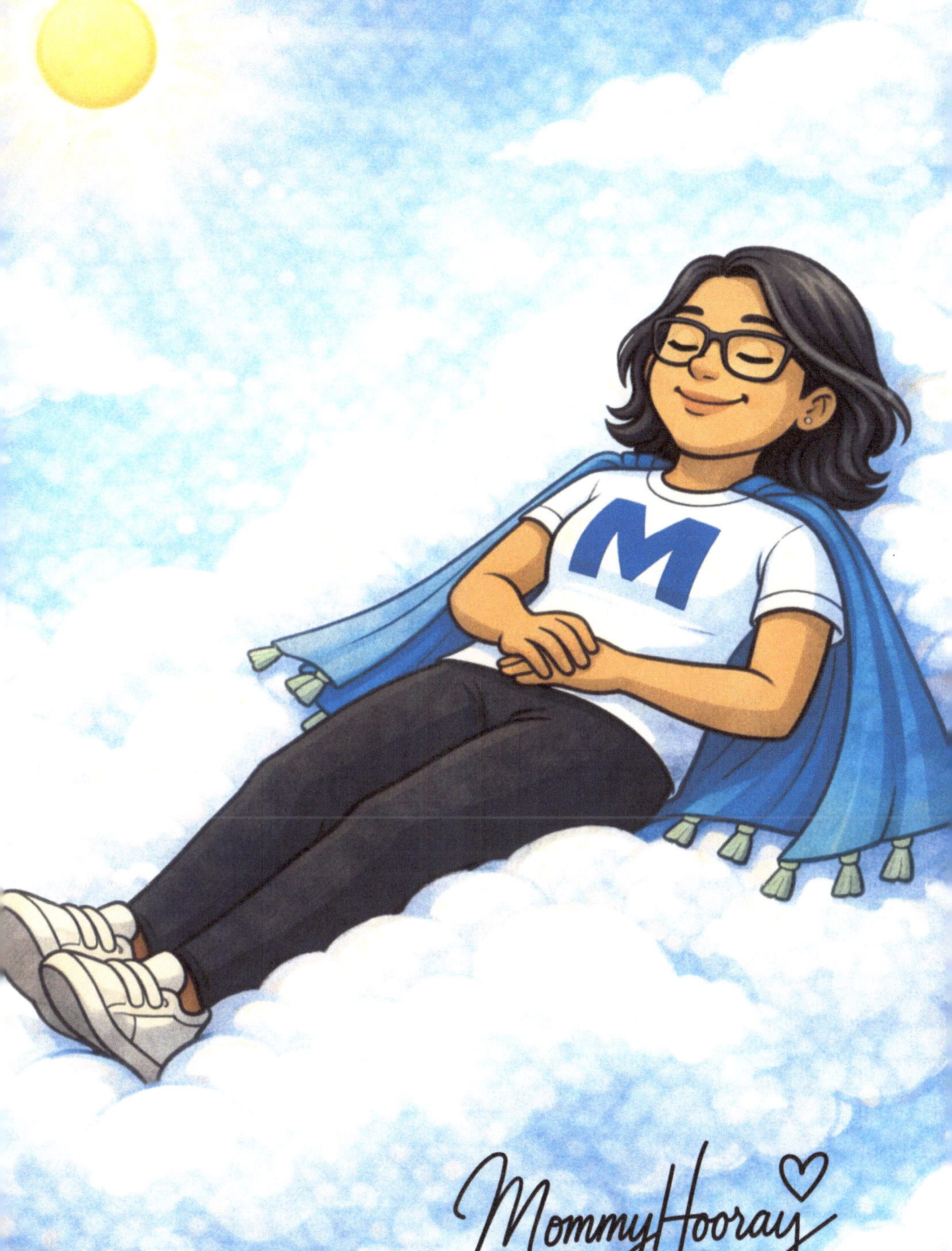
MommyHooray

# Also by MommyHooray

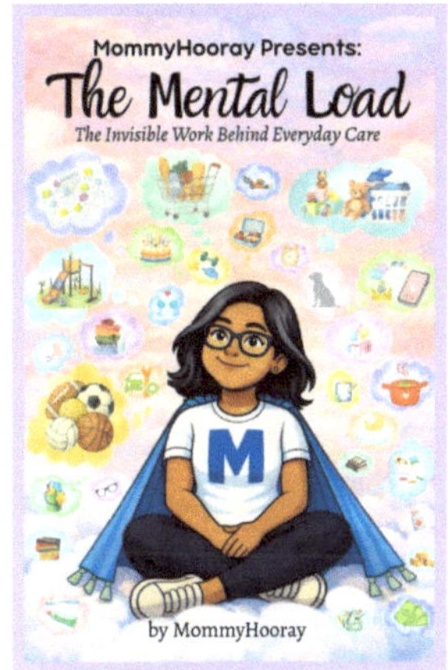


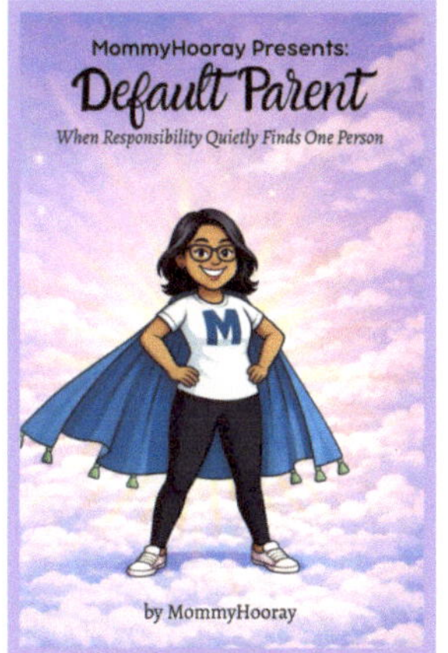


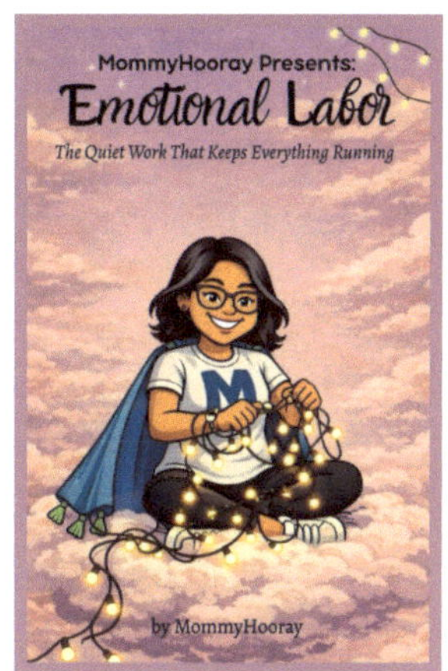


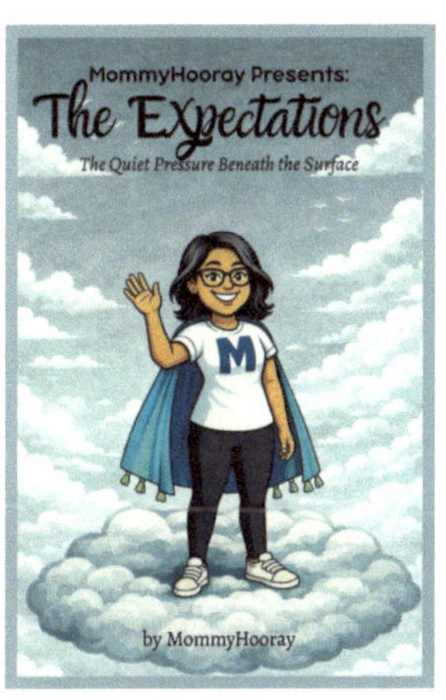


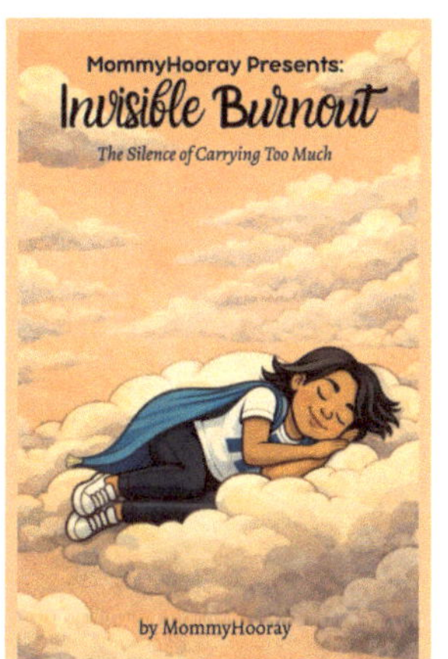


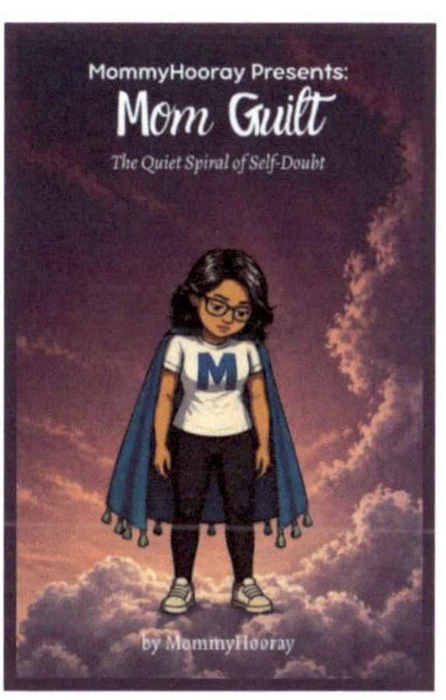


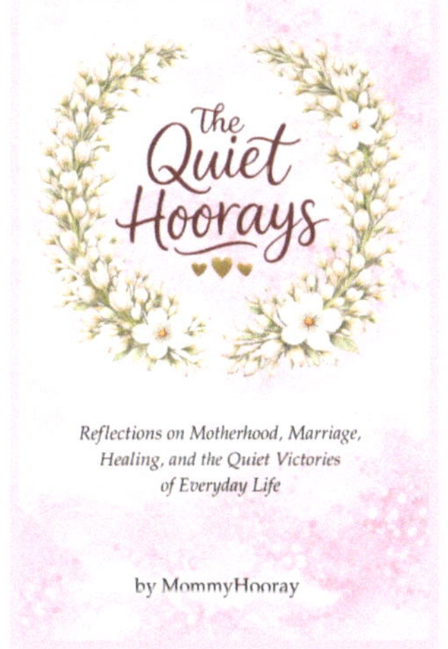


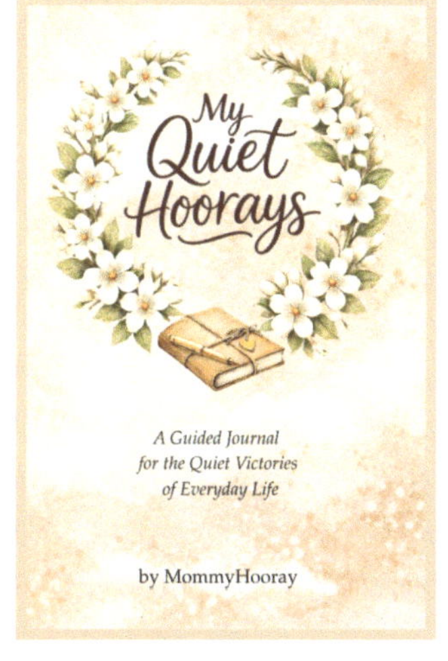


**... and more!**

# From My Heart to Yours

*Write something meaningful*
*for the person who will cherish this book, or for yourself.*

Today's Date: ________________

*May this page find you again, years from now.*

www.ingramcontent.com/pod-product-compliance
Lightning Source LLC
LaVergne TN
LVHW052300100826
845147LV00001B/98

* 9 7 8 1 9 7 2 0 7 1 4 1 0 *